Peppermint Oil

Everything You Need To Know About This Energizing Essential Oil

By Amy Joyson

The trademarks that are used are without any consent, and the publication of the trademark is without permission or backing by the trademark owner. All trademarks and brands within this book are for clarifying purposes only and are the owned by the owners themselves, not affiliated with this document.

Disclaimer – Please read!

The information provided in this book is designed to provide helpful information on the subjects discussed. This book is not meant to be used, nor should it be used, to diagnose or treat any medical condition. For diagnosis or treatment of any medical problem, consult your own physician. The publisher and author are not responsible for any specific health or allergy needs that may require medical supervision and are not liable for any damages or negative consequences from any treatment, action, application or preparation, to any person reading or following the information in this book. References are provided for informational purposes only and do not constitute endorsement of any websites or other sources. Readers should be aware that the websites listed in this book may change.

Table of Contents

Introduction

Peppermint Essential Oil is the second in the *Essential Oils Uncovered* series. This series of books will focus upon individual essential oils, the history, health benefits, and applications of each. In addition readers will be guided through the process of removing the oil from the plant, and the methods of processing the oil for each application. General application guidelines will also direct the reader through the use of essential oils for a variety of treatments. Historically essential oils have been an integral part of humanity. They have been used to treat many conditions and ailments. This work will discuss the historical uses of the essential oil, rediscovery of the use of essential oils, the modern adaptations, and potential future applications of the oils.

Peppermint essential oil is one of the earliest essential oils used medicinally. The oil was used by Egyptians, Greeks, and Romans, and during the middle ages. Many treatments using peppermint oil have been quite successful over the course of millennia. The modern era has taken up the mantle and continued using peppermint essential oil, in some cases as it was used in the ancient world. Fortunately scientific inquiry is catching up to what many have known- essential oils, and peppermint oil specifically, contains healing properties for a variety of ailments. Scientific research into essential oils has come a long way, proving what many have already known, and enlightening us further on the applications of peppermint essential oil for things we never before used it to treat.

One of the problems facing researchers when it comes to essential oils is the strength. As noted, the strength of essential oils can change based upon when the plant is harvested and how the oils is extracted. Uniformity is a necessary component for testing oils and their efficacy. Therefore reliable oil extraction is the key for any recipe using essential oil, just as in any investigation of essential oil. Whether you are harvesting your own oil, or purchasing oil, these factors must be taken into consideration. This work serves as template for peppermint essential oil use, based upon known cures, and the most recent scientific research into treatments using peppermint essential oil. As with all essential oils, a discussion on appropriate safety procedures is included. Heed the warnings and follow the instructions carefully for safest, healthiest treatments after consulting with your physician.

A History of Peppermint Essential Oil

The Egyptians and Greeks provide our earliest material evidence regarding the uses of peppermint in the ancient world. Although peppermint was not differentiated specifically from 'mint', peppermint was the strong mint that grew wild in Europe and easily was distinguished from soft mints like pennyroyal. Early mention of the mint appears in discussions of the God Hades, who was about to engage in a tryst with a river nymph Minthe, when Prosepine (Persephone) arrived and turned Minthe into a plant to be trampled underfoot. Hades took pity on his former lover and granted her the strong, sweet smelling properties that none could ignore. Since that time 'Minthe' (mentha) became the genus of the hundreds of varieties of mint in existence. Peppermint wasn't deemed 'pepper' mint in antiquity, and was just known as 'mint' (mentha) not unlike Hades' mistress. The abundance of the European peppermint plant along with excellent descriptions, historical accounts, and extensive studies tell us that most of the 'mint' denoted in the ancient medical texts are classified under the genus mentha piperita (peppermint.) Many believe that peppermint is a hybrid cross between spearmint and watermint, although that assumption is currently under scrutiny.

Historically, not all treatments using peppermint were essential oils. Some ancient recipes called for leaves steeped in hot water, like a tea, while others called for the extraction of the oil from the plant and infusion into other oils or liquids. As the distillation process was developed over the course of centuries, peppermint essential oil also became a target of the distillation process by the middle ages. This provided an opportunity for a stronger concentration of oils to treat a variety of ailments. Over the course of millennia, the uses of peppermint as a treatment changed due as much to experimentation and experience as creativity.

The Ebers Papyrus, a medical papyrus dating to 1500 BCE, noted that the Egyptians used mint to cure myriad ailments including flatulence, vomiting, and halitosis. The Egyptians were not the only ancient society to discover the health benefit of mentha. Mentha was so valuable to the Egyptians; it was often used as a form of currency.

The Greeks were well known for their treatment of disorders with many practitioners willing to record their treatments for history. Hippocrates noted the benefits of mentha to relieve headaches. There are substantial recipes included in the Hippocratic Corpus that involve peppermint. Some were quite reliable, while others appeared to be desperate attempts to relieve vexing ailments. Many Greeks used strong mint as an offering to Aphrodite to secure lustful desires, and strong mint was often associated with a heart's yearning in the ancient world.

The Romans also partook of the healing qualities of peppermint. Pliny discussed peppermint at length and mentioned wines made of peppermint and rue. He detailed the use of mentha as a good liniment. He discussed the use of peppermint for the expulsion of afterbirth, but noted that it was fatal to a fetus if taken before birth. Further conversation on peppermint by Pliny focused on the menthol component of peppermint as it soothed the voice, and healed the chaffing of the skin. For Pliny it was also a cure for cholera.

Another notable Roman medical practitioner, Celsus noted that peppermint was excellent for those that needed to increase their urine output. He wrote that this strong mint should be gargled to ease paralysis of the tongue. A draught of peppermint was taken for a moist cough if mixed with almonds and starch. Although not the same recipe Pliny also noted the efficacy of mint for cough. Strong mint was also recommended by Celsus for indigestion, and a vapor of peppermint for treatment of ulcers in the nostrils. Most notably, Celsus recommended a remedy of strong mint, endive and pomegranate mixed with cold water and a touch of wine to stop vomiting. This was confirmed by Pliny.

Ahmed Ibn al-Jazzar was a notable Muslim physician in the 960's CE. Al- Jazaar mentioned strong mint as a cure for erectile dysfunction, as well as a reliable treatment for kidney, liver, and intestinal diseases. Other medieval doctors also used strong mint to treat intestinal discomforts and aid in wound healing. It was during the Middle Ages that we see an increase in mint sauces and jellies, as mint was known to ease the digestion between courses and after meals. This was a time when Europeans were heavily influenced by Islamic cuisine and spices.

An early modern herbalist, John Gerard took up the mantle of recommending peppermint as a curative for hiccups. Gerard also suggested taking peppermint for mitigating nausea. Nicholas Culpepper was a noted herbalist during the colonial period and worked diligently to identify and inform his readers of not only what plants looked like, but how they might be used for healing and daily life. He noted that peppermint eased headaches, and soothed skin lesions and scabs. Culpepper also stated that nothing worked better to ease disorders of the stomach and intestines. As with previous medical writers, he suggested a poultice of peppermint to stop lactation and mentioned that it was excellent in fomenting the progress of childbirth. His recommendations for use suggested adding peppermint oil to water or distilled oil for best results.

Li Shih-Chen wrote a compendium of Chinese herbal medicine in the late 16th century and stated that peppermint oil was an antispasmodic. Clearly, the effects of peppermint on the gastric tract were known throughout history, and carried forward over the course of the ages. Native Americans used peppermint in a tea to alleviate gas pains. Colonists commonly added peppermint to pea soup to calm the stomach and aid digestion. The benefits of peppermint were recognized worldwide. Acres of peppermint were planted in Europe and the United States by the turn of the 20th century. The plant was desired for use by many for everything from culinary flavoring to healing remedies.

By the 1930's, scientific study was undertaken by internal medicine specialists with regard to peppermint, and the widespread use of mentha piperita as a household remedy. Verification of the effectiveness of peppermint essential oil as an antispasmodic and aid to other gastric issues was detailed. As medical schools began to take shape in the late 19th and early 20th centuries, a slow turn away from traditional herbal medicines was witnessed in the western world. Sadly, science was not as focused on the use of essential oils, as it was on surgical techniques and what many considered more 'modern' treatments.

Fortunately the world has turned back toward its roots once again and embraced herbal treatments. Many have always understood the benefits of herbs like peppermint, and science is finally beginning to catch up. Many research studies have gotten underway in the past two decades to begin to quantify through methodological scientific analysis, the properties, benefits, and risks of essential oils like peppermint. In many cases, this has served to verify what we have known for millennia, peppermint essential oil has abundant uses to humanity to heal, gratify, and flavor, just as it always has.

Peppermint Oil Extraction

The most common method of extracting oil from peppermint plants is distillation. The peppermint plant contains essential oils in the leaves, with very little in the flowers. Stems should be discarded and only the leaves should be used. Ideally dry, warm weather will yield more essential oils from the peppermint leaves. Gather the leaves immediately after bloom and distill while fresh for best results. Leaves should be free of major imperfections, washed, and allowed to dry.

Steam distillation is the most common form of distillation for peppermint leaves. This requires the use of a still, cooling tank (condenser) and oil separator. The chopped or macerated leaves should be placed on a grid or grate inside of the still. Steam should be directed into the still through the bottom. The high pressure and temperature will break through the plant cells containing essential oils. The steam and the oils will rise up and into the pipe that will carry them through the condenser where the oil and water are cooled. The cooled oil and water vapor will move into the oil separator. The oil is then siphoned off of the top while the condensed water can be released from the bottom.

An alternative to steam distillation is known as **Hydro-Diffusion**. Hydro-Diffusion forces steam into the top of the still, which reduces the distillation time. The steam and the oil will still rise into the pipe, and move into the condenser. The cooled oil and water vapor will move into the oil separator, as with steam distillation, to allow the oil to be siphoned off of the top.

Another method of extracting peppermint essential oil includes **Steam and Water Distillation**. This process is similar to steam distillation but generally results in a lower concentration of essential oil. Water is place in the bottom of the still. A grate or grid is located above the water. The macerated plant material is placed upon the grate/grid. As the water boils, the steam breaks down the plant cells. The oil and water vapor will be carried to the condenser to cool, and eventually separate as it reaches the oil separator. The oil will be siphoned off as with previous methods.

Peppermint Oil Preparation

Essential oils that are topically applied should be diluted first, as they are too volatile to be applied directly to the skin. Cold pressed base oil is optimal. Often Jojoba oil is used as a base for peppermint essential oil. Other base oils can also be used contingent upon individual preference, allergies, and applications. The standard method of determination of dilution is 1 drop of essential oil per 1 teaspoon of base oil is a 1% dilution, 2 drops of essential oil to 1 teaspoon of base oil is a 2% dilution, and so on. Different applications require different dilutions. Dilute accordingly. Please consult the 'General Guide to Applying Essential Oil' chapter for further details on carrier oils.

*Peppermint Infused Oil** is not an essential oil. This is referenced only for readers to discern and understand the difference. Infused oil comes from the mottling of freshly picked herbs into oil, and allowing that oil to sit is sunlight for three weeks. The oil is strained and then added once again to fresh herbs, repeating the process. A final straining of the herb material results in oil that has been infused with peppermint (or another herb). This is not essential oil, as the process does not allow for the breaking down of cells to release the essential oil. Infused oil does not contain the strength of constituents necessary for the treatment of ailments covered in this work.

The Key Properties of Peppermint Essential Oil

Peppermint has been documented since the first written language systems evolved around the Mediterranean region. This enduring and abundant mint has served as a flavoring, medicine, and aesthetic component to a host of rituals and cultural symbols. To address the longevity of peppermint in human history, it is necessary to examine the component structure of mentha piperita.

Peppermint contains a variety of active properties. Menthol is one of the primary constituents along with menthone, isomenthone, and methyl acetate. The secondary constituents in peppermint include alpha-myrcene, apha-caryophyllene, carvone, and pulegone. Additionally, mentha piperita has been found to contain trace elements of alpha-pinene, menthane, sabinene, terpinolene, alpha-terpinolene, ocimene, and fenchone. A determination of the concentration of these constituents and which of the lesser components may be present in peppermint is reliant upon when the peppermint is harvested, what parts of the plant are used, and how it is extracted. The optimal time to harvest peppermint is immediately after the bloom of the flower, when it is hot and dry. At this time the most essential oil can be found within the leaves, at greatest strength. See the chapter on extraction of essential peppermint oil for further details.

In examining what this means for those considering treatment with peppermint essential oil, a quick examination for those not versed in chemistry is necessary. Peppermint oil contains menthol, which has many health benefits that will be discussed throughout this treatment, but is also toxic in large doses. In addition, mentha piperita contains vitamin A, vitamin C, beta-carotene, folates, potassium, and iron. Peppermint also contains trace amounts of calcium, magnesium, and phosphorus. Rosmarinic acid, an antioxidant, has also been found in mentha piperita. These are all valuable vitamins and minerals to the human body, offering many health benefits to those partaking of peppermint. More detailed information on the specific health benefits is provided for the reader through the course of this work.

The Health Benefits of Peppermint Essential Oil

The health benefits of peppermint have long been known, from the ancient world to the modern day. It is only recently however that science has been able to more conclusively support this ancient household remedy. Since antiquity, peppermint has been known to relieve gas pain, and cure minor stomach ailments. Over the course of time, peppermint essential oil took on many other uses from cough and congestion relief to a cure for tennis elbow. Additionally, Vitamins C and K along with the primary constituents (including menthol) all serve to nourish or aid in healing of the body. In what capacity can the body be aided with peppermint essential oil?

As scientific research has been undertaken on essential oils in recent decades it has shed light upon the scientific reasons peppermint essential oil is an effective remedy for so many ailments. First and foremost, mentha piperita has been scientifically proven to be an antispasmodic agent. Historically this supports the use of peppermint essential oil to aid various stomach disorders, cure the hiccups, and ease coughs. In the modern world, doctors add peppermint essential oil to barium solutions to relax the colon during barium enemas. Doctors also administer enteric-coated capsules of peppermint essential oil to patients suffering from Irritable Bowel Syndrome (IBS). Scientific studies have demonstrated that 79% of IBS patients treated with enteric-coated peppermint essential oil capsules found relief from the abdominal pain, and 56% of those were completely pain free. Long term results show that overall, 57% of patients treated with enteric-coated peppermint essential oil capsules for IBS continue to demonstrate less abdominal pain and greater relief from symptoms, with limited side effects unlike many other IBS treatments. This is why peppermint essential oil is the first line of treatment doctors recommend for IBS patients. The antispasmodic properties of mentha piperita have also been established in tests conducted on surgical patients to mitigate post operative nausea and vomiting. The results have confirmed the efficacy of administering peppermint essential oil to those patients.

Peppermint essential oil has also been associated with oral health ranging from fresh breath to incorporation in toothpaste and mouthwashes. Scientifically, peppermint essential oil has verified antiseptic and antibacterial properties, explaining its inclusion in many oral hygiene applications. More recently peppermint essential oil was studied for effectiveness as an intracanal antiseptic solution against oral (bacterial) pathogens during root canals. Peppermint essential oil demonstrated significant antimicrobial effects. Further testing has established that peppermint essential oil attacks and stops the growth of antibiotic- resistant bacterial strains of some pathogens like helicobacter pylori and MRSA.

For millennia, peppermint has been used in poultices for the skin for a host of ailments from wounds, to rashes, to infections. The antiseptic and antibacterial agents in mentha piperita have also been examined, and well documented with regard to wound healing capabilities. This can be beneficial for almost anyone, but special focus for researchers concerned wound healing in those with diabetes, since they have greater difficulty healing on their own. The results are promising.

As mentioned, peppermint essential oil has been proven to aid other skin conditions. Commonly used to treat poison ivy and poison oak, the menthol in peppermint essential oil cools and soothes the rash, providing relief to the itching caused by histamine. Current research has conclusively found that peppermint essential oil also relieves symptoms of pruritus. This itchy skin condition has myriad causes from dermatitis to cancer treatments, but relief has been found with peppermint essential oil. Studies involving treatment of pruritus in pregnant women has been ongoing, but caution has been exercised in these studies due to the potential side effects of peppermint essential oil on pregnant females.

Mentha piperita has more recently been investigated with a focus on the antiviral properties. The focal point of testing has been against herpes simplex virus types 1 and 2. The results were promising, as concentrations of peppermint essential oil clearly demonstrated virucidal effects, which increased with the concentration of the oil. Further testing has been ongoing, and the best delivery method in treatment has yet to be determined. The antiviral properties of peppermint essential oil are also being carried out against Human Immunodeficiency Virus (HIV) with similar virucidal results. Although the peppermint essential oil acted as an antiviral against both viruses without destroying the cells, further testing is necessary to determine concentration and delivery. The results portend great progress in the treatment of a variety of viruses using mentha piperita.

Peppermint essential oil has achieved the reputation over the centuries as a certain cure for headaches. Research supports the effects of peppermint essential oil when used in combination with ethanol on headache symptoms, decreasing sensitivity while increasing the ability to concentrate. This provides a reliable alternative to drug therapies often used to treat chronic headaches without the limiting side effects of medication. There may be one additional benefit to the head from peppermint essential oil- hair growth! Studies comparing mentha piperita to monoxidil (standardly used in the treatment of hair loss) demonstrated that peppermint essential oil had a 92% hairgrowth rate (compared to 55% for monoxidil) without the damaging side effects. Scientists have concluded that peppermint essential oil facilitates hair growth by promoting the conservation of vascularization of the dermal papilla, resulting in rapid hair growth.

Peppermint essential oil also demonstrates antisoporific properties. It is quite common to experience periods of sleepiness during the day. Peppermint is an invigorant; a stimulant that can be used to combat the afternoon lull and provide the motivation to focus and keep working or playing each day. It also demonstrates improved cognitive functioning, a pleasant and most welcome side effect. When it comes to play, mentha piperita may also provide even greater benefits. Many athletes struggle with the desire to increase their performance without resorting to harmful chemicals to enhance results. Peppermint may provide the solution. Recent studies were conducted on healthy male athletes using an oral .05% solution of peppermint essential oil in a dilution of 500ml of mineral water. A baseline (pre-peppermint essential oil) of respiratory rate, blood pressure, oxygen, power, exertion, etc. was taken on each subject to map changes over a ten day period of administration of the mentha piperita solution. The results were conclusive, peppermint essential oil demonstrated the effective increase in exercise performance according to all tested (respiratory function variables, systolic blood pressure, heart rate, and respiratory gas exchange) parameters. The mechanisms behind the success of menthe piperita on exercise performance are still being studied.

The antioxidant potential of peppermint essential oil has also been oft discussed. The most recent research into the antioxidant properties of menthe piperita however is inconclusive. There is a demonstration of antioxidant capacbilities due to the rosmarinic (phenolic) acid contained within peppermint essential oil coupled with the strong presence of monoterpenes. The potential of these constituents is reliant upon many factors, from soil and climate harvested, to method of extraction, and synergistic compounds added. Although results show promise, there remains no firm methodology established with which to harvest, extract, and administer peppermint to act primarily as an antioxidant.

There are many potential uses for peppermint essential oil in treatment of a variety of conditions. Peppermint essential oil shows great potential in combating the spread of prostate and lung cancers, but testing is ongoing. Fortunately the scientific community has demonstrated an eagerness to unlock the potential of essential oils.

General Guide to Applying Essential Oils

Essential oils can be used to treat an immense variety of conditions. They provide a wonderful alternative or supplement to traditional medical treatments. Consult a physician before treatment of any condition and prior to the administration of any essential oil. Always follow all safety instructions provided before use of any essential oil. Also, check not only for drug interactions, but photo toxicity. These can be severely damaging. Always conduct a skin patch test prior to the administration of any essential oil whether for topical or oral use. Do not used expired essential oils, as with all organic material, essential oils have a viable shelf life. Using these oils beyond the expiry date can be hazardous to your health.

Read instructions thoroughly at least twice before preparation of the essential oil. This will prevent any mistakes in measurements, and offer optimal results for treatment. In addition be certain to know the strength of the essential oil. Many essential oils are sold as 100% pure, but are already diluted in a solution. This is typical, but critical to understanding what amount you will need to add/adjust to any solution, poultice, etc. If it does not state on the jar, ask. Many essential oil producers provide a standard dilution of their essential oils. Verify that you are indeed using essential oil, not extract or infused oil. Extracts and infused oils provide far different concentrations of essential oil constituents compared to pure essential oil. This will affect treatment protocols and may hinder results dramatically. Additionally, inquire as to whether the essential oil has been adulterated in any way. Some suppliers add synthetic chemicals to extend shelf life, or reconstitute the oil. Sometimes essential oils will not be purely from one species of plant, but a combination of similar plants. This too will affect any treatment protocol planned, and may cause an unwanted reaction. Much of this can be resolved by establishing a relationship with a reliable supplier of essential oils.

Application of essential oils usually falls into a few categories. Baths, poultices, inhalations, massage, and diffusion, are the most common. Oral administration is extremely rare and should only be undertaken with medical supervision, as serious complications may result. Essential oils are often added to baths for treatment of a variety of muscular aches and pains. Essential oils can irritate the skin, and should be used cautiously in a bath, as the effect can be systemic.

Carrier Oils

For the majority of treatments, essential oils are added to carrier oils. This is particularly true of 'hot' oils like peppermint, clove, cinnamon, lemongrass, etc. which need a carrier oil to protect the skin. Carrier oils come in many varieties, and should be chosen according to safety, interaction with the essential oil (if any), and skin sensitivity. The most common carrier oils are:

Jojoba Oil

Coconut Oil

Sweet Almond Oil

Olive Oil

Sesame Oil

Vitamin E Oil

Lanolin Oil

Shea Butter Oil

Shea Butter (raw form is fine for many remedies, depending upon the treatment)

In addition to this list, there are many other carrier oils like grape seed, and various nut oils (peanut, walnut, sunflower, etc.) Caution is suggested when using these oils as skin interactions are more likely with nut oils. Sesame oil, sweet almond oil, and Shea butter appear on the above list, as they offer the least reactivity of all the nut oils. If the patient already has a known nut allergy, it is recommended that non-nut based carrier oils are used. Oils like grape seed oil have low yields and often toxic solvents are used to pull enough of the oil from the seed, frequently leaving the toxic solvent (Hexane) in the extracted oil. This can be damaging with extensive or long term use. As with essential oils, it is always recommended to conduct a patch test before use to determine sensitivity to the oil. Some oil allergies require two separate applications before reactivity is experienced.

Those who are familiar with other books in this aromatherapy series will recall an earlier discussion of some of the techniques that may be used to apply essential oils for therapeutic purposes. Book number two, in particular, was entirely focused on one of these potential application methods – massage. However, there are many other methods through which essential oils may be administered to a patient.

Topical application

This is one of the most simple and direct methods for introducing an aromatherapy treatment. It requires very little technical skill; the applicant merely needs to determine *what* to apply to the body of the recipient, and *where* to apply the treatment for best results. When applied to the skin, the fine molecules of which essential oils are comprised permeate the dermis and enter the blood stream, circulating their therapeutic effect throughout the body. As a rule, topical application of essential oils should only be administered in diluted concentrations as the volatile compounds in some essential oils may cause an adverse reaction in some patients. However, due to the mild nature of lavender oil, it may be applied 'neat' in some special cases (although only under the direction of a trained aromatherapy professional). Some ways to topically apply essential oils include via self-application, massage, or diluted in bath water.

Massage

Massage is a great way to introduce essential oil treatment to an individual. It combines all of the advantages of topical application, with the added therapeutic benefits associated with massage itself. What's more, there are a number of very different massage techniques that can yield various benefits and treatment outcomes. For example, there is the basic 'Swedish' massage, the meditative 'raindrop technique' massage, as well as a number of other types that have a specific treatment focus (such as 'lymphatic drainage massage', for example). Massage can be a great way to induce relaxation, lower blood pressure, and treat muscle soreness, and can be used to complement the treatment aims of aromatherapy itself. Further to the topic of safety covered in the previous chapter, care should be taken to avoid massage treatment in patients who are experiencing acute illness (including those with fever), have open wounds or communicable disease, or tumours. Extreme care should also be taken when practicing massage with children and the elderly. If in doubt as to whether massage treatment will be appropriate for a given patient, seek the advice of a physician.

Those interested in a more in depth exploration of the used of massage in aromatherapy should consult the second book in this series, which is devoted to a thorough investigation of this art.

Inhalation

Inhalation can be a most suitable delivery method when it comes to aromatherapy treatment, for a number of reasons. First, it is one of the less invasive treatment options, as inhalation of the vapour of essential oils generally results in few complications for a patient. Second, inhalation takes advantage of the special aromatic qualities of essential oils, and the effect that they have on the body's limbic system. The limbic system is often referred to as the 'ancient' part of the brain. That is, it is one of the most primeval parts of the human anatomy, and is responsible for influencing much of basic human function as a result. Emotions, behavior and other rudimentary and atavistic psychosomatic processes are connected to and governed by the limbic system. The neural mechanism responsible for governing the brain's scent detection system (the olfactory system) is considered a part of the limbic system. Also included in the structure of the limbic system are the *hippocampus* (which plays a key role in the management of memories), the *nucleus accumbens* (responsible for reward, pleasure and addiction), and the *amygdala* (which controls the body's fear/stress response). Subsequently, the exposure of this system to aromatic essential oils can have a profound effect on these various primal functions.

Inhalation can be carried out in a few ways, but is typically split between *direct* and *indirect* inhalation methods. The former can involve, for example, the application of essential oils to a blank personal inhaler, or the addition of a few drops of oil to a steam basin. Indirect methods of inhalation focus on the general diffusion of essential oils and typically make use of some kind of whole room diffuser.

Ingestion

Perhaps the least common form of delivery of aromatherapy treatment, ingestion is nonetheless a suitable option in some cases. Some milder essential oils may be taken in this way when used in highly diluted concentrations. Lavender, for example, may be taken in specific cases as a circulation boosting cordial, or tonic. However, because of some of the risks of adverse reaction when it comes to orally administering essential oils (such as severe irritation of the digestive system), this type of treatment is best left to the remit of trained professionals. One should therefore, avoid taking or administering essential oils through this method as a general rule.

Complete Safety With Peppermint Essential Oil

As with all essential oils it is necessary to take precautions for health and personal safety. Always consult a physician before beginning any course of essential oil treatment. Consultation is a critical step to correctly diagnose the problem the essential oil is intended to treat. Additionally, it is vital to discuss with a physician any plans to treat a condition with essential oil for possible drug interactions, allergies, and other counter indications.

Peppermint essential oil offers many health benefits in the treatment of a variety of ailments. It can however be dangerous when used improperly, or by those with certain conditions. Please read these safety precautions carefully before beginning any treatment plan:

1) Peppermint essential oil should NEVER be used by pregnant women. Essential oils can cross the placental barrier and reach the child. Additionally, as with many members of the mint family, peppermint is contraindicated during pregnancy as it may contribute to pre-term labor, or miscarriage since it is a known emmenagogue.

2) Peppermint essential oil should NEVER be used by lactating women, as it will cause the milk to dry up.

3) Peppermint essential oil should NEVER be used on children under the age of 6 years old, as menthol (a primary ingredient in peppermint) has been known to arrest breathing in children. It is also known to cause jaundice in babies with a G6PD deficiency (causing red blood cells to die.)

4) People with gall bladder inflammation, liver disease, hiatal hernia, gastroesophogeal reflux, or obstruction of the bile ducts should not use peppermint essential oil as it is may contribute to the aggravation and worsening of these conditions.

5) For cancer patients taking 5-Fluorouracil, peppermint essential oil can increase skin absorption of the drug. It is extremely important to discuss the use of peppermint essential oil with your oncologist before administration.

6) Those patients taking Felodipine for high blood pressure, or the immunosuppressant Cyclosporine should consult a physician before use of peppermint essential oil as it increases the bioavailability of the drugs. This allows the drugs to remain in the body longer than anticipated and may be dangerous.

7) Those patients with diabetes should consult a physician before use as Peppermint essential oil may lower blood sugar levels, resulting in hypoglycemia.

8) Peppermint essential oil should not be used topically on the face, near the eyes, nose, or mouth.

9) Caution should be exercised with the use of peppermint essential oil as it has been known to irritate the mucous membranes when inhaled.

10) As with all essential oils, a skin patch test should be conducted to determine sensitivity, and allergies. Apply a single drop of peppermint essential oil (diluted with 1 teaspoon of carrier oil –Jojoba, Almond, or Coconut) directly on the wrist. Wait 24 hours without washing. If a reaction is present, do not use the peppermint essential oil in any treatment. It is recommended that a test of the carrier oil be

carried out prior to testing the peppermint essential oil for an accurate determination of sensitivity.

11) Potential side effects of peppermint essential oil use:

> -Nausea

> -Anorexia

> -Contact Dermatitis (when used topically)

> -Hypersensitivity Reactions

12) As with many essential oils, taking more than the prescribed amount can be toxic. Menthol is toxic in large doses, and as a primary constituent of mentha piperita, extreme caution should be used. Always consult a physician before use.

13) Volatile essential oils like peppermint should always be stored in a cool, dry place to retain the strength of the constituents contained therein.

14) Do not use essential oils beyond the stamped expiry date as this may be harmful.

15) Essential oils should never be applied to the genitals.

Pure Peppermint Essential Oil Remedies

Ailment 1: Irritable Bowel Syndrome (IBS)

Treatment: Take 1 (.2 ml) enteric coated capsule of peppermint essential oil 3 times per day.

Warning: Taking peppermint essential oil that is not contained in an enteric coated capsule will aggravate symptoms of Irritable Bowel Syndrome. The enteric coating is a protectant and the only successful way to administer peppermint essential oil for the treatment of Irritable Bowel Syndrome. The enteric coating prevents release of peppermint essential oil in the stomach, allowing release in the intestine. This is optimal for successful treatment without irritation. Consult with your physician before administration.

Ailment 2: Headaches

Treatment: Dilute 1 drop of peppermint essential oil into 1 teaspoon of jojoba or coconut (carrier) oil. This is a 1% solution and should be used for anyone with sensitive skin. Gently rub diluted essential oil onto temples. It may also be applied to the back of the neck for localized headaches. Repeat every 3 hours as necessary.

A 2% dilution (2 drops of peppermint essential oil per teaspoon of carrier oil) is only indicated for those that have used a 1% dilution without reaction, and minimal results were achieved.

Warning: Keep peppermint essential oil away from the eyes, nose, and mouth. Do not exceed a 2% dilution as skin irritation will result. Always skin test any essential oil and carrier oil before application.

Ailment 3: Congestion

Treatment:

a) Place 3-5 drops of peppermint essential oil into an essential oil diffuser. Do not hold your face close to the essential oil as it is emitted from the diffuser. Breathe in through the nose.

b) Add 3 drops of peppermint essential oil into a ceramic or metal bowl of boiled, distilled water (that has cooled slightly). With a towel draped over the head, lower face towards the bowl (about 12 inches) and inhale through the nose slowly for about 10 minutes, or until the congestion has eased. It is highly recommended that an eye protectant (mask) is worn, as peppermint essential oil can irritate the eyes.

c) Apply 2 drops of peppermint essential oil onto a handkerchief. Hold handkerchief in the palm of the hands and lower face 1-2 inches from handkerchief, inhaling through the nose. Repeat 3 times per day to ease symptoms.

d) Apply 2 drops of peppermint essential oil onto a cotton ball. Waft under the nose while inhaling through the nose. Repeat 3 times per day to ease symptoms.

Ailment 4: Fever

Treatment:

a) Mix 2 drops of peppermint essential oil with 1 teaspoon of carrier oil (jojoba, coconut, or almond oil is recommended). Massage this solution gently along the spine.

b) Relief can also be found by adding 1 drop of peppermint essential oil to 1 teaspoon of carrier oil. Rub gently across the forehead, temples, soles of feet, and back of neck.

Warning: Keep away from the eyes. Always skin test any essential oil and carrier oil before application.

Ailment 5: Nausea, motion sickness

Treatment:

a) Place 3-5 drops of peppermint essential oil into an essential oil diffuser. Do not hold your face close to the essential oil as it is emitted from the diffuser. Breathe in through the nose.

b) Mix 1 drop of peppermint essential oil with 1 teaspoon of carrier oil. Rub directly and gently onto abdomen.

c) Add 1 drop of peppermint essential oil to 1 teaspoon of honey. Add 1 cup of hot water. Allow to cool (enough to sip.) Sip slowly until nausea subsides. Repeat in 3 hours if necessary.

d) Place one drop of peppermint oil on the tongue and hold to the roof of the mouth an hour before travel.

Warning: Do not use treatment **c** or **d** if you have acid reflux or irritable bowel syndrome as this will worsen symptoms. Please read safety instructions chapter for other conditions* that may be affected.

Ailment 6: Cough

Treatment: Mix 1 drop of peppermint essential oil with 1 teaspoon of carrier oil. Gently rub onto the chest. Breathe normally. Repeat 2 times per day if necessary.

Warning: Always skin test any essential oil and carrier oil before application.

Ailment 7: Tendinitis (wrist, elbow, shoulder, ankle)

Treatment: Mix 5 drops of peppermint essential oil to 1 teaspoon of carrier oil. Rub gently into skin near affected tendon. Apply twice per day.

Warning: Always skin test any essential oil and carrier oil before application. This recipe is particularly strong*

Ailment 8: Muscular Pain

Treatment: Add 10 drops of peppermint essential oil to 1 tablespoon of jojoba oil. Massage firmly but not vigorously into affected area daily.

Warning: Always skin test any essential oil and carrier oil before application.

Ailment 9: Gas Pain/Bloating

Treatment:

a) Add 1 drop of peppermint essential oil to 1 teaspoon of honey. Add 1 cup of hot water. Allow to cool (enough to sip.) Sip slowly until nausea subsides. Repeat in 3 hours if necessary.

b) Mix 1drop of peppermint essential oil with 1 teaspoon of carrier oil. Rub directly and gently onto abdomen.

Warning: Do not use treatment **a** if you have acid reflux or irritable bowel syndrome as this will worsen symptoms.

Ailment 10: Foot Odor

Treatment: The antifungal and antibacterial properties of peppermint essential oil are extremely beneficial in the treating the causes of foot odor, along with the refreshing, pleasant aroma.

a) Add 10 drops of peppermint essential oil to a foot bath. Soak feet for 10-15 minutes. Dry. Repeat 2-3 times per week.

b) A drop of peppermint essential oil may be added to each shoe to help keep bacteria (and consequently odors) at bay.

c) Add 10 drops of peppermint essential oil to 1 tablespoon of coconut oil. Massage firmly onto feet and on and between toes. This may be repeated 3- 5 times per week as necessary.

Warning: Always skin test any essential oil and carrier oil before application.

Ailment 11: Halitosis

Treatment: Add 3 drops of peppermint essential oil to 1 cup of cold water. Add 1 teaspoon of baking soda. Shake vigorously. Swish/gargle mixture in mouth for 2 minutes. Discharge mixture. Mouthwash can be stored in a cool dry place. The anti-bacterial properties aid in alleviating the causes of halitosis.

Warning: Do not swallow*

Ailment 12: Energize and Focus

Treatment: Peppermint essential oil has long been known to invigorate the mind and body to provide focus.

a) Apply 2 drops of peppermint essential oil to a handkerchief. Place handkerchief in palm of hand and inhale through the nose.

b) Apply 2 drops of peppermint essential oil onto a cotton ball. Waft under the nose while inhaling through the nose.

c) Apply 3-5 drops of peppermint essential oil into an essential oil diffuser.

d) Mix 1drop of peppermint essential oil with 1 teaspoon of carrier oil. Apply to shoulders and back of neck.

Ailment 13: Wound healing, eradication of bacteria

Treatment: Mix 1 drop of peppermint essential oil with 1 teaspoon of olive oil. Apply a small amount to the wound. Repeat 2 times per day for 1 week. Mixture May also be applied to a cloth, and then applied to the wound, if sensitive. Keep wound clean and open to allow wound to breathe and heal.

Warning: Always skin test any essential oil and carrier oil before application.

Ailment 14: Hair Growth (and Hair Health)

Treatment: Mix together thoroughly 3 drops of peppermint essential oil with 1 teaspoon jojoba oil (add 3 drops of Vitamin E oil for sensitive skin.) Rub onto scalp daily to promote hair growth, stop dandruff and odors. This recipe can be doubled for large scalp areas. Begin treatment 2 times per week. This may be increased to three applications per week.

Warning: Keep mixtures away from the eyes, as it is an irritant.

Ailment 15: Sunburn Relief

Treatment: Mix together 3 drops of peppermint essential oil with 2 tablespoons of lanolin oil (this is effectively acting as the moisturizing carrier oil and acts to prevent the drying or burning sensation on the skin). Apply to affected area. Substitute carrier oils such as olive or jojoba oil are extremely suitable as well. Apply twice per day.

Warning: Always skin test any essential oil and carrier oil before application.

Ailment 16: Asthma

Treatment: Apply 3 drops of peppermint essential oil onto a cotton pad. Inhale normally through the nose for 10 minutes. Repeat 3 times per day to ease symptoms.

Ailment 17: Pruritus, hives, poison oak, poison ivy, bug bites

Treatment: Combine 6 drops of peppermint essential oil with 1 ounce of sesame oil (coconut oil can be easily subsituted.) Apply two times per day to the affected area for two weeks.

Warning: Always skin test any essential oil and carrier oil before application.

Ailment 18: Critter Ridder -to rid your home of mice, rats, and unwanted creepy crawlers

Treatment:

a) Mix 60 drops of peppermint essential oil with 8 ounces of water. Add a drop of plain dish detergent to mixture for blending purposes. Shake well and place inside of spray bottle. Spray areas inside of home where critters and crawlers may gain access, or have taken up residence, once per week.

b) Add 3 drops of peppermint essential oil to cotton balls. Place cotton balls in areas where critters and crawlers are known as well as any potential access points. Cotton balls must remain dry to be effective. Replace cotton balls 1-2 times per week as needed.

Ailment 19: Hiccups

Treatment: Place 2 drops of peppermint essential oil onto a cotton ball. Waft under the nose, breathing in normally. Repeat if necessary.

Ailment 20: Stress Relief

Treatment: Place 5 drops of peppermint essential oil into a diffuser. Breathe normally. The peppermint essential oil acts to calm the central nervous system and reduce stress.

Ailment 21: Rheumatoid Arthritis/ Arthritis

Treatment: Add 40 drops of peppermint essential oil to 3 ounces of sesame oil. Let rest for one week in a cool, dark place. Rub several drops on hands and feet daily as needed. Mixture may be applied to other joints with arthritic pain as well. Store mixture in a cool, dry place in the dark.

Warning: Always skin test any essential oil and carrier oil before application.

Remedies Using 100% Pure Peppermint Essential Oil Blends

Ailment 1: Sunburn

Treatment:

a) Combine 2 drops of peppermint essential oil with 1 drop of lavender essential oil. Add that to 1 tablespoon of jojoba oil and 1 tablespoon of lanolin oil. Apply to affected area twice per day.

b) Combine 2 drops of peppermint essential oil with 1 drop of lime essential oil (steam distilled as cold pressed results in photosensitivity). Add to 2 tablespoons of lanolin oil. Apply to affected area twice per day.

Warning: Always skin test any essential oil and carrier oil before application.

Ailment 2: Wound healing, eradication of bacteria

Treatment:

a) Combine 2 drops of peppermint essential oil with 2 drops of eucalyptus essential oil and 2 drops of lavender essential oil. Add to 1 cup of warm water. Soak clean, dry gauze in mixture and apply to clean wound. Let rest 15-20 minutes and remove. Allow air to circulate and wound to dry. Repeat 3 times per day.

b) Combine 2 drops of peppermint essential oil with 2 drops of lime essential oil (steam distilled as cold pressed results in photosensitivity) and 2 drops of lavender essential oil. Add to 1 cup of warm water. Soak clean, dry gauze in mixture and apply to clean wound. Let rest 15-20 minutes and remove. Allow air to circulate and wound to dry. Repeat 3 times per day.

Warning: Always skin test any essential oil and carrier oil before application.

Ailment 3: Cough

Treatments:

a) Mix 1 drop of peppermint essential oil with 1 drop eucalyptus essential oil and 1 teaspoon of olive oil. Gently rub onto the chest and back. Breathe normally. Repeat 2 times per day if necessary.

b) Add 3 drops of peppermint essential oil, 2 drops eucalyptus essential oil to essential oil diffuser. Breathe normally through the nose.

Warning: Always skin test any essential oil and carrier oil before application.

Ailment 4: Congestion

Treatments:

a) Add 2 drops of peppermint essential oil and 2 drops of rosemary essential oil into a ceramic or metal bowl of boiled, distilled water (that has cooled slightly). With a towel draped over the head, lower face towards the bowl (about 12 inches) and inhale through the nose slowly for about 10 minutes, or until the congestion has eased. It is highly recommended that an eye protectant (mask) is worn, as peppermint essential oil can irritate the eyes.

b) Apply 1 drop of peppermint essential oil and 1 drop eucalyptus essential oil onto a handkerchief. Hold handkerchief in the palm of the hands and lower face 1-2 inches from handkerchief, inhaling through the nose. Repeat 3 times per day to ease symptoms.

c) Apply 1 drop of peppermint essential oil and 1 drop eucalyptus essential oil onto a cotton ball. Waft under the nose while inhaling through the nose. Repeat 3 times per day to ease symptoms.

d) Mix together 2 drops of peppermint essential oil, 2 drops eucalyptus essential oil, and 1 drop rosemary essential oil with 1 tablespoon carrier oil. Massage gently on chest and back. Apply twice per day as necessary.

Warning: Always skin test any essential oil and carrier oil before application.

Ailment 5: Asthma

Treatments: a) Add 2 drops of peppermint essential oil and 2 drops of eucalyptus essential oil into a ceramic or metal bowl of boiled, distilled water (that has cooled slightly). With a towel draped over the head, lower face towards the bowl (about 12 inches) and inhale through the nose slowly for about 10 minutes, or until the congestion has eased. It is highly recommended that an eye protectant (mask) is worn, as peppermint essential oil can irritate the eyes.

b) Add 2 drops peppermint essential oil and 2 drops lavender essential oil to a handkerchief. Hold handkerchief in the palm of the hands and lower face 1-2 inches from handkerchief, inhaling through the nose for 10 minutes.

c) Combine 8 drops peppermint essential oil, 20 drops eucalyptus essential oil, and 28 drops lavender essential oil. Add 5 drops of the mixture into an essential oil diffuser. Inhale normally.

Ailment 6: Tendinitis (wrist, elbow, shoulder, ankle)

Treatment:

a) Mix 10 drops of peppermint essential oil with 10 drops rosemary essential oil and 10 drops Roman chamomile essential oil to 2 tablespoons of coconut oil. Rub gently into skin near affected tendon. Apply twice per day.

b) Mix 10 drops of peppermint essential oil with 10 drops rosemary essential oil and 10 drops lime essential oil (steam distilled as cold pressed results in photosensitivity) to 2 tablespoons of coconut oil. Rub gently into skin near affected tendon. Apply twice per day.

Warning: Always skin test any essential oil and carrier oil before application. This is a very potent remedy.* Chamomile is not suggested for use on those with ragweed sensitivity.

Ailment 7: Critter Ridder -to rid your home of mice, rats, and unwanted creepy crawlers

Treatments:

a) Mix 40 drops of peppermint essential oil and 20 drops of hyssop essential oil with 8 ounces of water. Add a drop of plain dish detergent to mixture for blending purposes. Shake well and place inside of spray bottle. Spray areas inside of home where critters and crawlers may gain access, or have taken up residence, once per week.

b) Add 2 drops of peppermint essential oil and 2 drops hyssop essential oil to cotton balls. Place cotton balls in areas where critters and crawlers are known as well as any potential access points. Cotton balls must remain dry to be effective. Replace cotton balls 1-2 times per week as needed.

Ailment 8: Nausea, motion sickness

Treatments:

a) Place 3 drops of peppermint essential oil and 2 drops lavender essential oil into an essential oil diffuser. Do not hold your face close to the essential oil as it is emitted from the diffuser. Breathe in through the nose.

b) Mix 1 drop of peppermint essential oil and 1 drop lavender essential oil with 1 teaspoon of almond oil. Rub directly and gently onto abdomen.

c) Combine 2 drops of peppermint essential oil to 2 drops ginger essential oil and 5 drops olive oil. Rub 8 drops of mixture onto chest and abdomen at least one hour prior to travel.

Warning: Always skin test any essential oil and carrier oil before application.

Ailment 9: Headaches

Treatment:

a) Combine 1 drop of peppermint essential oil and 1 drop lavender essential oil into 1 teaspoon of almond oil. This is a 2% solution, and is strong. It should not be used for anyone with sensitive skin. For those with sensitive skin, add another teaspoon of almond (or jojoba) oil to the mixture. Gently rub diluted essential oil onto temples. It may also be applied to the back of the neck for localized headaches. Repeat every 3 hours as necessary.

b) Mix 1 drop of peppermint essential oil and 1 drop lime essential oil (steam distilled as cold pressed results in photosensitivity) into 1 teaspoon of jojoba oil. This is a 2% solution, and is strong. It should not be used for anyone with sensitive skin. For those with sensitive skin, add another teaspoon of almond oil to the mixture. Gently rub diluted essential oil onto temples. It may also be applied to the back of the neck for localized headaches. Repeat every 3 hours as necessary.

Warning: Always skin test any essential oil and carrier oil before application.

Ailment 10: Seasonal Allergies

Treatment: Mix together 10 drops peppermint essential oil, 10 drops lemon essential oil, and 10 drops lavender essential oil with 2 tablespoons olive oil. Place a few drops of the mixture onto hands and rub bottoms of the feet, the back of the neck, and the forehead. Place hands together and slowly, deeply inhale. Repeat twice per day as needed.

Warning: Always skin test any essential oil and carrier oil before application.

Ailment 11: Irritable Bowel Syndrome (IBS)

Treatment: Combine 2 drops hop flower essential oil (humulus lupulus) and 2 drops peppermint essential oil with 1 tablespoon coconut oil. Rub a half teaspoon of the mixture on the abdomen. Repeat 2-3 times per day as needed. Mixture should be stored in a cool, dark place.

Warning: Always skin test any essential oil and carrier oil before application.

Ailment 12: Hot Flashes

Treatment: Add 2 drops peppermint essential oil, 2 drops lemon essential oil, and 1 drop clary- sage essential oil to 1 tablespoon olive oil. Rub a few drops on the temples, chest, and lower back

Warning: Always skin test any essential oil and carrier oil before application. Keep away from eyes, nose, and mouth as this is an irritant.

Ailment 13: Menopausal symptoms

Treatment: Mix 2 drops peppermint essential oil, 1 drop Roman chamomile essential oil, 1 drop clary-sage essential oil, 6 drops lemon essential oil, 5 drops geranium essential oil with 1 ounce lanolin oil and 1 ounce raw Shea butter. Combine well. Massage into fatty areas of the body on a daily basis. Estrogen becomes specific to adipose tissues after menopause, and is targeted specifically with this treatment. The treatment may be used over the whole body if desired, but is not necessary.

Warning: Always skin test any essential oil and carrier oil before application. Chamomile is not suggested for use on those with ragweed sensitivity.

Ailment 14: Gas Pain/Bloating

Treatment: Add 2 drops Roman chamomile essential oil, 2 drops peppermint essential oil, and 1 drop orange essential oil to 1 tablespoon olive oil. Apply to abdomen and massage gently.

Warning: Always skin test any essential oil and carrier oil before application. Chamomile is not suggested for use on those with ragweed sensitivity.

Ailment 15: Fevers

Treatment:

a) Combine 1 drop peppermint essential oil, 1 drop wintergreen essential oil and 1 teaspoon jojoba oil. Rub on temples, back of neck and soles of the feet.

b) Combine 1 drop peppermint essential oil, 1 drop lime essential oil (steam distilled as cold pressed results in photosensitivity) and 1 teaspoon jojoba oil. Rub on temples, back of neck and soles of the feet.

Warning: Always skin test any essential oil and carrier oil before application.

Ailment 16: Energize and Focus

Treatment:

a) Place 3 drops peppermint essential oil and 2 drops lemongrass essential oil into an essential oil diffuser. Breathe normally.

b) Combine 1 drops of peppermint essential oil with 1 drop lemongrass essential oil and 1 teaspoon coconut essential oil. Apply in a gentle massage to shoulders and back of neck.

c) Place 1 drop each of peppermint and lime essential oils into a handkerchief. Place handkerchief in palm of hands and slowly inhale through the nose.

d) Place 1 drop each of peppermint and lemongrass essential oils onto a cotton ball. Waft cotton ball under nose.

Warning: Always skin test any essential oil and carrier oil before application.

Ailment 17: Head Lice

Treatment: Combine 5 drops peppermint essential oil, 6 drops ginger essential oil, and 5 drops lavender essential oil with 1 tablespoon walnut oil. Massage thoroughly into scalp and hair. Wrap head in a towel overnight. Repeat nightly until lice is eradicated.

Warning: Always skin test any essential oil and carrier oil before application. Keep out of eyes, nose and mouth as these are known irritants.*

Ailment 18: Heartburn

Treatment: Mix 1 drop of peppermint essential oil with 1 drop angelica essential oil and add that to 1 teaspoon coconut oil. Rub on upper abdomen, repeat every 2 hours as necessary.

Warning: Always skin test any essential oil and carrier oil before application. Angelica is a photoxic essential oil. Keep skin out of sub/tanning beds after use.

Ailment 19: Stress Relief

Treatments:

a) Place 3 drops peppermint essential oil and 2 drops ylang ylang essential oil into a diffuser. Breathe normally.

b) Place 3 drops peppermint essential oil and 2 drops lemongrass essential oil into a diffuser. Breathe normally.

c) Place 2 drops peppermint essential oil and 2 drops angelica essential oil into a diffuser. Breathe normally. The peppermint essential oil acts to calm the central nervous system and reduce stress.

Ailment 20: Arthritis/ rheumatoid arthritis

Treatments:

a) Mix together 45 drops of peppermint essential oil with 15 drops yarrow essential oil and 3 ounces sesame oil. Let rest for one week in a cool, dark place. Rub several drops on hands and feet daily as needed. Mixture may be applied to other joints with arthritic pain as well. Store the mixture in a cool, dry place in the dark.

b) Combine 40 drops of peppermint essential oil with 10 drops rosemary essential oil and 10 drops lavender essential oil. Add to 1 ounce jojoba oil, and 2 ounces almond oil. Let rest for one week in a cool, dark place. Rub several drops on hands and feet daily as needed. Mixture may be applied to other joints with arthritic pain as well. Store the mixture in a cool, dry place in the dark.

Warning: Always skin test any essential oil and carrier oil before application.

Conclusion

Peppermint essential oil (menthe x piperita) has been scientifically proven to be an invaluable resource for myriad ailments. It has been well documented that peppermint essential oil does possess many of the healing and nutritive properties the ancients claimed. The remedies contained within this book are the best available to treat the conditions covered. Some treatments may provide greater relief than others, depending upon not only the severity of the condition, but also the individual. Each individual must find what works best for them. Sometimes allergies, other precipitating conditions, or medications may play a role in the sensitivity and effectiveness of the remedies.

Science has taken up the mantle of researching the effectiveness of not only peppermint essential oil, but many more essential oils for the purposes of providing another avenue of treatment for the body, mind, and spirit. Thank you for taking the journey of healing with peppermint essential oil. This was only the second book in the *Essential Oils Uncovered* series. Please join us for the next step on the healing journey, *Frankincense Essential Oil.*

Check Out My Other Essential Oils Books!

Simply click on the books title or type the links below into your web browser. Alternatively you can search for "Amy Joyson" in the Kindle Store.

Essential Oils: The Complete Guide:
http://www.amazon.com/gp/product/B00T12QLW4

Essential Oils Massage Techniques:
http://www.amazon.com/gp/product/B00VITFIQI

Essential Oils For Allergies:
http://www.amazon.com/gp/product/B00X6ANQKM

Essential Oils For Dogs:
http://www.amazon.com/gp/product/B00XSDE6N8

Lavender Essential Oil:
http://www.amazon.com/gp/product/B00WTBTHPC

2 FREE eBooks for you!

Guys, thanks so much for reading my book. I truly hope it served as a great introduction to lavender essential oil. As a token of appreciation I have prepared two free ebooks for you. Here is a bit of information about them!

The 10 Most Important Essential Oils

In this book we delve deep into the uses and applications of the ten essential oils that I consider to be the most 'essential'. For each oil I explain the key health benefits, teach you the therapeutic applications and provide specific safety precaution. I include one of my most useful remedies for each of the oils as well. So you will receive a deep knowledge of ten essential oils and ten brilliant remedies for free! It is a 10k word eBook, the same length as this one!

When you receive this ebook you will also receive a couple of emails from me a week containing even more information about the essential oils! I will endeavour to give you at least 5 recipes or remedies per week and also provide you with some great information on the lesser known essential oils.

Type this link into a web browser: http://bit.ly/1EuHgyn

The Ultimate Guide To Vitamins

This is another wonderful 10k word ebook that has been made available to you through my publisher, Valerian Press. As a health conscious person you should be well aware of the uses and health benefits of each of the vitamins that should make up our diet. This book gives you an easy to understand, scientific explanation of the vitamin followed by the recommended daily dosage. It then highlights all the important health benefits of each vitamin. A list of the best sources of each vitamin is provided and you are also given some actionable next steps for each vitamin to make sure you are utilizing the information!

As well as receiving the free ebooks you will also be sent a weekly stream of free ebooks, again from my publishing company Valerian Press. You can expect to receive at least a new, free ebook each and every week. Sometimes you might receive a massive 10 free books in a week!

Type this link into a web browser: http://bit.ly/1EuHgyn

About The Author

Hey there! I'm Amy Joyson, a lifelong student of holistic and alternative medicine. My journey began as far back as I can remember, my mother, a practicing aromatherapist, taught me value of natural remedies as a youngster. I don't think I could imagine a life without the essential oils if I tried, they are just so important to me. I am passionate about sharing their value with as many people as possible, which led me to writing my books. If you have read any of my books I truly hope they have added value to your life and I thank you with all my heart for trusting in me.

Outside of being an author, I work as a personal trainer. Employing my deep knowledge of alternative treatments has enabled me to provide outstanding results for all of my clients!

In my spare time you will often find me lounging in my hammock reading the latest aromatherapy magazine or romantic fiction novel. I have a soft spot for true romance! I aim to meditate at least once a day, and practice yoga 5 times a week. My biggest hobby however is exploring the beautiful world that we live in. Next on my hit list is Iceland, there is something seriously alluring about that island.

Valerian Press

At Valerian Press we have three key beliefs.

Providing outstanding value: We believe in enriching all of our customers' lives, doing everything we can to ensure the best experience.

Championing new talent: We believe in showcasing the worlds emerging talent by giving them the platform to grow.

Simplicity and efficiency: We understand how valuable your time is. Our products are stream-lined and consist only of what you want. You will find no fluff with us.

We hope you have enjoyed reading Amy's guide to Peppermint Essential Oil

We would love to offer you a regular supply of our free and discounted books. We cover a huge range of non-fiction genres; diet and cookbooks, health and fitness, alternative and holistic medicine, spirituality and plenty more.

You can type this link into your web browser:

http://bit.ly/18hmup4

Free Preview of "Lavender Essential Oil"

Lavender oil is derived from the steam distillation of the plant of the same name (typically, the *Lavandula angustifolia* species of the lavender genus), which is believed to be native to the Mediterranean region of Southern Europe and North Africa. Lavender is classified as a flowering herb and is a member of the mint family. It has enjoyed its position as a revered medicinal herb for some thousands of years, with evidence of popular use in nearly all major ancient Eurasian cultures. The Ancient Egyptians are known to have used lavender in the preparation of tinctures for use during the embalming process, while it was also found to be a key ingredient in the herb, spice and sawdust blend used to stuff mummies and aid with their preservation. Additionally, lavender was commonly used in Egypt in various cosmetic preparations. The Greeks also used lavender prolifically, however, their usage of the flower took on a more therapeutic bent than the Egyptians. There, the plant was used as a cure-all remedy for various psychosomatic conditions, from insomnia to insanity and beyond. The contemporary name for the plant is possibly derived from the Latin *lavare*, or 'to wash', which hints at the typical Roman usage of the flower. (Another potential etymological source comes from the Latin word *livindulo*, meaning 'livid or bluish'). Typically, lavender was used as an aromatic by the Romans to scent their baths, dwellings and clothing. Lavender was also used cosmetically by wealthy patricians throughout the Empire as a perfume and treatment for the skin and hair.

Whatever the true origin of the present day name of the plant, lavender has maintained a long association with cleanliness and purification, from ancient times through to the modern era. There is an abundance of evidence of a strong connection between domestic cleanliness and the usage of lavender as a purificant across cultures; here again, the etymological connection is clear. The word 'launder' is believed to have evolved from *lavendre*, which is the Old French word for the same term. Indeed, the use of lavender in instilling freshness in clothing and linens via special lavender infused washes was a common practice used by 'launderers' throughout history, with evidence of this practice existing across a number of different cultures. The appeal of lavender for use as a cleaning agent is certainly understandable; not only does the strong, yet pleasant scent of the flower mask any potentially offensive odors, but fabrics (and flesh) treated with lavender would have been noted to have kept cleaner for a longer period than those effects and persons treated without it. This would have seemed like a rather magical property in pre-modern times; however, we now know this attribute is due to the antimicrobial effect of lavender, which would work to kill bugs that generated nasty smells.

Yet, it is not merely the power of lavender to clean that has given this special plant such a revered place in history. The medicinal and healing properties of lavender have also long been observed and held in high esteem. We have already seen how the Ancient Greeks used lavender to treat various health related conditions. Interestingly, however, this tendency to use lavender for medicinal purposes is one that endured for centuries and was again a practice that permeated throughout various cultures. For example, grave robbers during the 17th century proliferation of the Bubonic Plague throughout France are rumoured to have maintained their good health (despite the extremely dangerous nature of their work) by washing in a powerful disinfectant known as 'Four Thieves Vinegar'. As one might expect, one of the principal ingredients in this prophylactic against one of history's deadliest diseases, was humble lavender. Though the narrative of this story likely has its foundations in folkloric mythology, there is colloquial evidence of lavender being used around this time to ward off the insidious 'Black Death'.

Lavender also has strong links to the modern foundation of the practice of aromatherapy. In fact, it is often viewed as the 'first oil' of the discipline, both in chronological and taxonomical terms. In the case of the former, it can be linked to a very particular moment in the history of aromatherapy, when Rene Gatefossé (a renowned French chemist) stumbled upon the remarkable healing properties of lavender oil. As with many great scientific discoveries throughout history, Gatefossé's encounter with lavender oil as an agent for healing was largely serendipitous. During an unrelated scientific experiment gone awry, the chemist received severe burns to his hands and arms. In a moment of desperation, he plunged his hands into the nearest available solution that could likely provide relief to his injuries – a large vat of lavender oil. Although Gatefossé is understood to have not been fully aware of the healing potential of lavender oil at the time, the remarkable qualities of the essence soon became apparent to him, as his injuries began to heal at an unexpectedly rapid rate. This experience soon saw Gatefossé begin a further scientific exploration of the therapeutic qualities of other essential oils. This eventually led the French chemist to become known as the 'father of aromatherapy', and one of the leading figures in driving a renewed interest in the remedial potential of essential oils in modern times.

However, it isn't simply because of its place in history that lavender is viewed with such pre-eminence in the world of aromatherapy. In taxonomical terms, there are many arguments for placing lavender oil at the top of the tree, especially when it comes to the oil's long list of remarkable therapeutic properties. As we have seen from the above historical accounts, lavender exhibits some very powerful antimicrobial qualities. Its prolific usage in cleaning and personal hygiene across various cultures is not coincidental; rather, the antibacterial effect of lavender that can help to kill bugs and germs is also effective in eliminating nasty odors. Additionally, its attribution as a key ingredient in the plague-fighting 'Four Thieves Vinegar' provides another hint at the oil's strong antimicrobial properties. While most modern users of lavender are unlikely to need to recruit lavender for use as a prophylactic against the Black Death, it nonetheless has a number of therapeutic applications for the remedy of a number of bacteria related complaints. Although its use as a prophylactic against disease in pre-modern times would perhaps have had more of a basis in mysticism than science, we know today that lavender can be relied upon as a powerful natural antiseptic. We will discuss all of these therapeutic attributes of lavender in more detail in later chapters.

As we can see from this brief introduction to lavender, perhaps no other oil has been more influential or remarkable in its consistent and common use among different cultures throughout history. Its range of uses has varied over time from disinfectant and deodorant, to antiseptic and relaxant, and many more. Today, lavender remains immensely popular, both for its unique fragrance and for its plethora of therapeutic qualities when used in aromatherapy treatments. With a broad understanding of the historical significance of lavender oil, we will take a detailed look in the following chapter at the properties that are responsible for bestowing such a mighty reputation upon this humble plant.

To grab this complete guide to lavender essential oil simply type this link into your web browser:

http://www.amazon.com/gp/product/B00WTBTHPC

Or search for Amy Joyson on Amazon!

Printed in Great Britain
by Amazon